Brains Over Brawn

By

Mark H. McCraw

This story is realistic fiction. I have recreated events, locations, and conversations from my memories of events in my life. In many instances, I have changed the names of individuals and places to keep their anonymity. I also have changed many identifying characteristics and details, such as physical properties, occupations, and places of residence. Any similarities are coincidental.

Contents

I dedicate this book to all the children or adults
who have ever been bullied.

Chapter 1:

Amid the Hurricane

My name is Marcus. The beginning of my story dates to my fifth grade. Shalimar, Florida, is my hometown. Shalimar, located in Florida's panhandle, has a population of approximately seven hundred people. People call it a panhandle because if you look at a map of Florida, you can see that the top of Florida looks like the handle of a pan. We lived in a two-bedroom, one-bathroom house on a cul-desac close to a swamp. There were tons of snakes where I lived. The proximity of the beaches was the best part of living here.

It takes around 45 minutes to reach the beaches of Shalimar. While Florida has beautiful beaches, living there comes with the risk of hurricanes that can wipe out property and homes.

June marks the beginning of hurricane season, which ends in September. Scientists name hurricanes after people in alphabetic order. Although hurricanes vary, our preparedness remains consistent.

Before Hurricane Eloise arrived, my dad boarded up the windows. We had to get ready emergency supplies such as rations, flashlights, water, and food. For safety measures, businesses and homeowners boarded up their buildings to prepare for the storms. I experienced Hurricane Eloise.

When the waves washed out the roads near the beaches, they would disappear into the Gulf of Mexico. Highway 98 is a coastal road that is over six hundred miles long in Florida that runs from south Florida to the panhandle of Florida.

On one side of the bridge on Okaloosa Island and Destin is a bay. The opposite side features the Gulf of Mexico and the beachfront. I love living in this area because it is so nice. Spring Break brings in a lot of tourists, which is a significant source of revenue for our town. Tourists always keep Fort Walton Beach, Okaloosa Island, Destin, Navarre, Pensacola, and Panama City bustling.

Boat owners during hurricanes should take their boats out of the water and put them in a dry dock, which is a large metal building. I used to think boats were stacked one on top of the other, but they sit on racks with space in between. I could not believe these racks could hold sailboats and other boats.

Trailer residents must move because of hurricane threats. To prevent destruction by high winds, military bases lock down and move airplanes. I loved seeing the weather planes flying around.

In anticipation of the hurricane, Dad would always instruct us to go to the hallway for protection against the fierce winds and force. He would say to stay away from windows because of possible flying glass. The high winds hitting our windows always scared me.

We used to listen to the weather on a portable radio during storms. In case of a power outage, we had flashlights ready. Hurricanes cause power outages. After the storm, we would assess the damage. Our property would occasionally experience fallen trees, broken windows, or flooding.

Hurricane Eloise caused damage to my grandfather's sailboat. The high winds picked up the sailboat, and the boat sank.

The dock building and the boats inside it were also damaged by the storm. Near the boat docks, waterspouts, which are like water tornadoes, were created. Hurricanes sometimes create these waterspouts and tornadoes.

My dad was fed up with the constant harsh weather. He worked as the manager of the Parts Department at a local dealership. Dad moved to New Hampshire to work at his friend's garage.

I felt frustrated and angry about moving because I had to leave my friends, but I had to obey my parents' orders. So, my family packed up all our belongings and moved to Kingston, New Hampshire.

Chapter 2:

The Long Trip

I had never been to the East Coast above North Carolina before. We were all squeezed into the moving truck during the long trip. We had all our possessions in the truck. The long trip made me nervous. The duration felt lengthy. We had a dog named Sandy, who was a brown Cocker Spaniel, but she passed away before we moved to New Hampshire.

During bathroom breaks, we came across rest stops that required a quarter for bathroom usage. I thought this was strange. In addition, I observed the Coke machines were pricier than in Florida. As we progressed up the coast, food prices increased. The weather in North Carolina was colder than I expected.

My childhood was spent in the panhandle of Florida, from first to fourth grade and later in junior high and high school. My foster grandfather Mel used to take us to Maggie Valley, North Carolina, which was the furthest I had ever gone. My birthplace is South Carolina, and I would visit my

Grandpa Mel's house there. Although I was an only child, I had five grandfathers, which I found impressive. I spent time with each one. As a young boy, I was fortunate in that regard.

I could not believe how busy New York City was while traveling through. The city is overwhelming with all the cars and people, and it is my first time experiencing it. When we crossed a bridge, I saw the Statue of Liberty.

Upon our arrival in Kingston, New Hampshire, the weather was cooler than in Florida and the scenery was beautiful. Since I came from the beach, I am accustomed to warm weather, so it will take me some time to adjust to this new climate.

My father's boss, his wife, and their kids hosted us. My dad had known these amazing people for a long time. It was helpful that my dad knew people up here as we transitioned to our new home.

Chapter 3:

Living with Friends

Eating together around the table is my fondest family memory. At least we had beds and great food to eat. Their house was enormous with many rooms in the house. Living with other families was difficult. Eventually, we resolved the situation.

The difference in accents between my family and our hosts made me feel strange. They did not appear to care, and neither did we. I was told to go to the "caw" once, but I did not know where that was. I requested additional information, and they referred to the "*car.*" We all laughed.

It was enjoyable to live with them and play with children my age. Our hosts were helpful as we integrated into New Hampshire. Dad found us a house in Peace, New Hampshire after we spent around a month at our host's house.

Chapter 4:

Our New Town

Peace, New Hampshire had a population of around 1,000, making it a small town. I was intrigued by the name of the town, as the name was unique and not like any other town name I had come across. Our house was situated around a mile from the school. Peace Elementary included students from kindergarten to eighth grade.

Starting at a new school in New Hampshire had me feeling apprehensive.

This town was rich in history, boasting a barrel factory, a house-turned-post office, a home with a grocery store on the bottom floor, an elementary school, and old, historic houses on Main Street. It seemed like the town only had one road, Main Street. Our residence was on Main Street, alongside other houses.

Exploring the town was my favorite activity. I had fun exploring the town on foot. The grocery store inside a house was unlike any other I had seen. I saw a huge turkey hanging in the store and informed my mom when I got home. I suggested we should get one for Thanksgiving.

Chapter 5:

Our New Home

Our home was a single-story house with an attached apartment and a wooden shed. Our house was enclosed by a chain-link fence. A narrow driveway was next to our house and opened onto Main Street. Our house was flanked by other houses on one side and across from us, while the other side boasted a vast field, giving me a view of the school a mile away.

When my dad purchased the house, there was a lady living in the apartment connected to our house. My dad allowed her to stay in the house while we were living there. The house we lived in had only one bedroom for my parents. My dad planned to build a windowless room for me in the center of the house, since I had no bedroom. Having a window would have been great, as my room was always dark. According to my dad, we modified the house for prior residents who were disabled because the counters were low. When we bought the house, we had to elevate the counters.

Our house had a nice fireplace and a basement that was home to our washer and dryer. Often used, the wooden stairs made spooky creaking sounds. The basement walls were constructed with granite. My mom believed the basement was haunted.

Our house had a second level that burned down twice in its history. A book was found by the tenant in our apartment that showed a deed for part of our property,

which was owned by a famous New Eng-
land poet. It was impressive to have a famous person as the previous owner of the
land.

Although winters are picturesque in Peace,
the snowfall was severe. The car needed to
be warmed up, and the driveway shoveled
before my dad could leave for work. Snow-
plows pushing snow into our driveway
were something I hated. Removing snow
was a physically challenging activity.

Did I ever tell you how much I hated it when the town snowplow pushed snow into our driveway, and we had to keep shoveling? Shoveling every day was our re-ality!

Chapter 6:

The Lady Next Door

Meeting our next-door neighbor at her house for the first time led me to believe that she possessed peculiar powers. She always was aware of my mom and dad's conversations. I could only think of her as a witch or a psychic. Another theory I had was that she had created tiny openings in the wall to eavesdrop. Even though it may sound weird, I thought she had a cauldron like the witches in movies. However, I was fond of the woman.

In my instances, I sometimes experienced loneliness in our new house, although I liked it. I feel like an outcast in this town because I do not have any friends. The surrounding people were mostly adults. I did not know any kids who lived in the neighborhood. The thought of meeting new people and having new experiences at the new school made me nervous.

When I was in Florida, I had three friends.

The absence of friends made it challenging

for me to settle in New Hampshire.

Chapter 7:

The Winter Holidays

Our winters felt like they would never end. Our summers were more like autumn because of the low temperatures. Winter, particularly during Christmas when it snowed, was my favorite time of year. Sitting next to a roaring fireplace with snow falling outside was mystical and impressive. If I am cold, the fireplace is my favorite spot.

Snow was a novelty to me since I only witnessed it once in Florida. My parents took me out for fun in the small amount of snow on the ground.

My dad had a snowmobile that I was eager to learn to drive. The snowmobile was huge. Riding it in the field next to our house was enjoyable until I hit a hill. Because of the sharp turn, the snowmobile flipped and fell on me. I will never ride a snowmobile again after this.

Going to Canada with his friend to ride snowmobiles was one of Dad's favorite things. I wanted to come along, but Dad refused to let me. He requested I stay and take care of my mom.

My mom had to work night shifts at a creepy nursing home. The haunted nursing home was a source of fear for my mom during her night shifts. She was assisting a blind and bedridden man on the second floor during one of her work nights. A wheelchair was said to have rolled across the resident's room. She was working with only one other nurse who was on the bottom floor, collaborating with another resident. My mom mentioned that this building was quite spooky.

Chapter 8:

Visits with Grandpa Mel

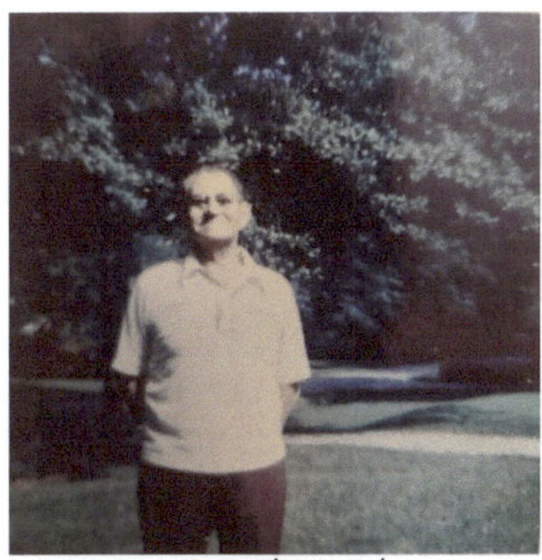

Grandpa Mel

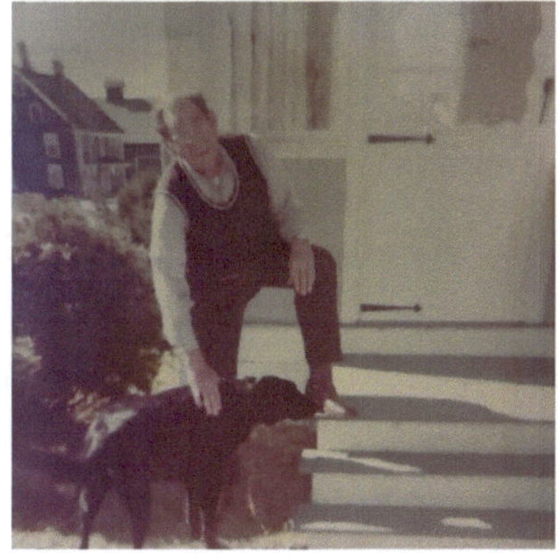

Grandpa Mel With A Neighborhood Dog

My grandpa from South Carolina came to visit us in New Hampshire for one month. Seeing him made me smile. Grandpa Mel stood at six feet, four inches tall and weighed around 240 lbs. My grandpa was not biologically related to me. My mom was adopted by him and Grandma. I loved him equally.

He was a World War II veteran responsible for operating heavy equipment such as bulldozers and overseeing military burials. During the war, the Army assigned him to work at Diego Garcia.

After the war, my grandfather became a prison guard for a chain gang in South Carolina. I can recall a time when I was three years old, and he took me through this place. The sight of inmates on their bunks, handcuffed to their beds as I walked past, scared me. Their faces looking at me are still fresh in my memory.

My grandfather often got ringers while playing horseshoes, showing his skill. It is a mystery to me how he did it. Because of cataracts, Grandpa had trouble seeing. Going to fish camps was one of his favorite things to do, which is equivalent to going to a seafood place in modern times. Fish camps are in the backwoods near Spartanburg, South Carolina. This is where I was born and holds significant memories for me. Grandpa's favorite activities included visiting peach factories, picking beans from farms, and bringing home corn on the cob in large bushels.

While at his house, I would walk down to the fence and receive money from his friend next door, which was always enjoyable. We went on trips together, including visits to Florida's theme parks.

Once, he desired a specific Christmas tree from a store. The only tree that captured his interest was the display tree with Christmas lights and decorations. Asking a store employee about it, he was told it was for display only. "No" was not an acceptable answer for my grandpa. He grabbed the Christmas tree, along with all its decorations, and paid before walking out the door.

Our server at a restaurant was not coming to the table, and I could not figure out why. Grandpa removed his dentures and left them in a glass of water on the edge of the table. I saw and said, "Grandpa!" I was in disbelief when I saw it. But it was my Grandpa Mel about which I am talking. He is incredibly important to me.

Chapter 9:

Mrs. C's Class

At Peace Elementary, my new school, the hallways were crowded and chaotic, with students ranging from K to eighth grade. My fifth-grade teacher was Ms. C. to me because her last name was hard to pronounce. The name was of Italian descent. I have a memory of her sitting a foot away from her desk, which I found odd. She was sincerely a gracious lady.

This unfamiliar environment made me feel strange. I stood out among other students because of my Southern accent. I had a one-of-a-kind voice that did not sound like anyone else. From the time I was new to the block, I have wanted to make friends.

Adjusting to such a momentous event as moving to a small historic town like Peace was challenging. When I left my only known home, I felt lost with no guidance during the transition.

Chapter 10:

My Bullies

I was a victim of bullying during my school days. Bullies used to chase me down the hallway to hit or yell at me. They were always together as a group. Because of my circumstances, I was unsure of how to manage a group of bullies who did not like me. My Southern accent or newness in town had something to do with it. I was too shy, which gave them the advantage.

Each day, I would feel nervous and reluctant to attend school the following day. To my mom, I would say that I was feeling sick.

This lasted for a long duration. Someone in town once shot at me with a BB gun and I got hit with a pellet after school. The bullying was happening without my parents' knowledge. My parents were clueless or believed I was always unwell.

Fear held me back from sharing with them. I regret not speaking up back then. Bullying, whether physical or verbal, was not a fun experience. Addressing the issue at school with my dad could have caused increased bullying.

What made other kids avoid playing with me? Regrettably, I had no friends except for those in Kingston. The small town was enjoyable for me. It would have been nice to have a friend.

Chapter 11:

Our Side Trips

I had to figure out how to bypass bully-ing. To distract me from bullying at school, Dad took us on small trips.

One time, we drove to Exeter, New Hampshire. Exeter was exciting because it contrasted with small and rural Peace, New Hampshire. It had power plants and nuclear plants in town.

We drove to the airport in Boston, Massachusetts during another trip. I could not figure out why we went to the airport. I believed my grandfather was coming, and we had to go pick him up. I would often experience car sickness when I was young. I fell ill in the airport bathroom after we stopped. After leaving, I caught sight of a popular football player who also acted in commercials.

As I saw him, he was running fast through the airport.

Small family trips were a distraction, but it was still too hard to forget about the kids who bullied me. I could not produce a way to put an end to their actions.

Chapter 12:

Mysterious Guest Speakers

During my time at Peace Elementary, we had the pleasure of hearing from guest speakers Mr. and Mrs. Hall. According to them, aliens abducted them.

The speakers that visited were the strangest I had ever encountered. While driving through a mountain pass, the Halls reported being abducted by aliens. They said that aliens beamed them up to their spaceship. Popularity of alien abductions and Unidentified Flying Objects (U.F.O's.) incidents were being reported as high during that time.

I did not believe them at first, but their stories were fascinating and helped me take my mind off the bullies. I questioned whether my classmates believed them.

Chapter 13:

The Special Event

The teacher announced that a spelling bee would be held for grades 5-8. The school-wide spelling bee involved the top three spellers from each grade. The winner of the school-wide spelling bee would take part in the regional spelling bee. The champion of the competition will advance to the national spelling bee in Washington, D.C.

I was thrilled about this chance. My teacher gave us a spelling book of words to memorize and study for the competition. My spelling skills were excellent, which is why I got involved. I could shift my attention away from constantly being bullied by other students, if nothing else. I concentrated on studying the Spelling book my teacher provided for the spelling competition. Every night, I would go home and study while memorizing the spelling words in the Spelling book. Several days after school, I would study my Spelling book at the library. The book was massive and overwhelming. There were three columns of words on every page. The fact that I could remember all of them before the spelling bee contest surprised me.

Chapter 14:

Brains Over Brawn

Instead of physically fighting back against the school bullies, I tried to outsmart them. I used my "brains over my brawn." This reminded me of my third-grade memory.

During third grade, my teacher had a jar with a "brain" in the classroom. It was fascinating finally to see a brain up close after never having done so before. The brain with giant wrinkles was gray. The brain was immersed in a liquid. The teacher's lecture always distracted me.

The body's brain is a dominant and remarkable part. Think of it as a control center that can do anything. I applied my mental capacity to win the spelling contest.

My victory resulted from my hard work and practice. I competed and won the school-wide competition, too! I was bursting with pride over my achievement!

The regional spelling bee competition is my next destination. The prospect of the regional spelling bee as a fun challenge had me excited. My determination and nightly studying left me eager to take on the next level.

Chapter 15:

Excitement Turned to Anger

My dad informed me one day that we were moving back to Florida. I was puzzled why. Was it because he did not enjoy the job? Was he not profiting at all? He kept the reason to himself.

He made me upset and angry when I had just won something important to me.

I succeeded because I was diligent, committed, and persistent. I believed it to be my first move towards fitting in.

The regional championship spot went to the spelling bee runner-up.

We lived in Peace for just a year before my dad took us back to Florida. We headed towards warmer weather.

Chapter 16:

The Lesson I Learned

What is the takeaway from my experience? My bullies stopped bothering me once I won the competition. Winning the spelling bee earned me the respect of my bullies. Outsmarting bullies was my strategy for overcoming their bullying. I used my "brains over my brawn" to stop them.

Overcoming them physically would have been easier, but I had too many bullies to manage solo. The reason behind their bullying will always be unknown to me. These were my reflections on the matter.

Being a fifth grader, I still chose not to engage in fights with others. It did not fit my style. I tried a different approach. Winning resulted from me using my brain.

Chapter 17:

Acting Out in Sixth Grade

I moved back to Florida during my sixth-grade year. During my time in Florida, I turned into a bully. When I look back, I feel regretful.

It all began on the playground when I knocked a girl's ball out of her hand while she was playing at recess. Once I was a playground bully until a bigger bully arrived and took over as king of the playground. My behavior was not good

when I heard we were moving back to Flor-

ida.

Chapter 18:

Becoming a Bully in Middle School

During my time in seventh and eighth grade, I frequently engaged in fights. Eventually, I grew tired of getting into fights and visiting the principal's office.

It was during Geography class after lunch when I would hear the office staff call my name over the intercom to report to the head office. Fighting was a common occurrence for me in the locker rooms, hallways, Commons Area, and school. I was disciplined by my teachers and coaches for misbehaving.

I was bullied by other middle school students during this time as well. Once, on the bus, I attempted to locate a seat. There was only one seat available, and it was next to a girl who was a ninth grader. She would not let me sit down and scratched my face with her long nails. I disliked this immensely. Even though my parents taught me to never hit girls, I felt like I had to because of what she did to me.

Chapter 19:

What I Would Do Now

As a child, the kids bullied me at the bus stop and my mom saw it happen. She told me to take care of them. My mom wanted me to defend myself. Bullies were not my thing, so I fought them.

In our world, not everyone can speak in a kind way to others and instead choose to bully others. The real problem is that not everyone will like you. What is important is that you like yourself and show kindness to others, which is difficult when you are being bullied.

I regret not reporting bullies earlier. It is so important. I wish I had reported my bullying in fifth grade. My mom was unaware until I became an adult. I am curious about how things would have changed if I had reported my bullies as a child.

Schools educate on preventing bullying. Putting bullying prevention lessons into practice is necessary for students. There are many strategies to manage bullies.

Chapter 20:

Types of Bullying

Can you define bullying? Bullying runs rampant in schools. "According to the U.S. Department of Human Health and Services, about 20 percent of students aged 12-18 experience bullying nationwide."

There are three common types of bullying, according to the Department of Health and Human Services:

- Verbal bullying is saying or writing mean things. Verbal bullying includes:

  - Teasing,
  - Name-calling,
  - Inappropriate sexual comments,
  - Taunting, or
  - Threatening to cause harm.

- Social bullying, sometimes called relational bullying, involves hurting someone's reputation or relationships. Social bullying includes:

  - Leaving someone out on purpose,
  - Telling other children not to be friends with someone,

- o Spreading rumors about someone, or
- o Embarrassing someone in public.

- Physical bullying involves hurting a person's body or possessions. Physical bullying includes:

  - o Hitting,
  - o Kicking,
  - o Pinching,
  - o Spitting,
  - o Tripping or pushing,
  - o Taking or breaking someone's things, or
  - o Making mean or rude hand gestures.[1]

---

[1] Source: www.stopbullying.gov.

Kids who are bullied can feel like they are:

- Different
- Powerless
- Unpopular
- Alone

Kids who are bullied have a hard time standing up for themselves. Bullying can make kids:

- Experience feelings of sadness, loneliness, or anxiety
- Feel physically sick
- Have problems at school
- Bully other kids.[2]

Social media platforms can also be a breeding ground for bullying through

---

[2] Source: www.stopbullying.gov

comments, videos, chats, Messenger, and other online communication methods. It is easy to respond to people on the internet. People have many ways to bully you online. Today, we call this "CYBER BULLYING."

The internet can be both useful and dangerous, so it is important to keep that in mind. Be careful! Bullying is a societal disease, no matter how you look at it. Bullying can occur between kids, but it also happens between adults.

The intention of bullies is to have the advantage. They exert their control over you. Your size, shape, nationality, speech, accent, physical appearance, perceived weakness, or age may make you a target. The motives behind bullying are the unknown. What drives them to do this? Analyzing everyone would be helpful in figuring this out.

We hold the ability to prevent bullies, and that is important to keep in mind. It is important to report bullies, since someone in authority can step in and halt their actions. When you are being bullied, physically or verbally, by a bully in class, ask your teacher to move you away from the bully. Hold your ground, do not yield. Do not give up and seek help.

Chapter 21:

Practicing Respect

Everyone should be treated with kindness. Respect is a powerful tool in treating people well. Treat people with respect by:

- Stopping and thinking before you say or do something that could hurt someone.
- Find something else to do. If you feel like being mean to someone, play a game, watch TV, or talk to a friend.
- Talking to an adult you trust. They can help you be nicer to others.

- Remembering that everyone is different and has unique experiences. It is not okay to bully people because they differ from you.
- Acknowledging your actions. If you think you have bullied someone in the past, apologize.[3]

---

[3] Source: www.stopbullying.gov

Chapter 22:

What Are Your Strategies
to Prevent Bullying?

Can you produce different strategies to halt bullying?

My intention in authoring this story was to provide you with new strategies for dealing with bullying. I have used resources from www.stopbullying.gov. It is a wonderful place to begin your research.

Work together with your parents or teachers to navigate this process.

Bullying is a universal phenomenon that has been exacerbated by social media. Do not forget that everyone is capable of being a bully. Our goal is to prevent bullying and spread respect and kindness in a world that deserves it.

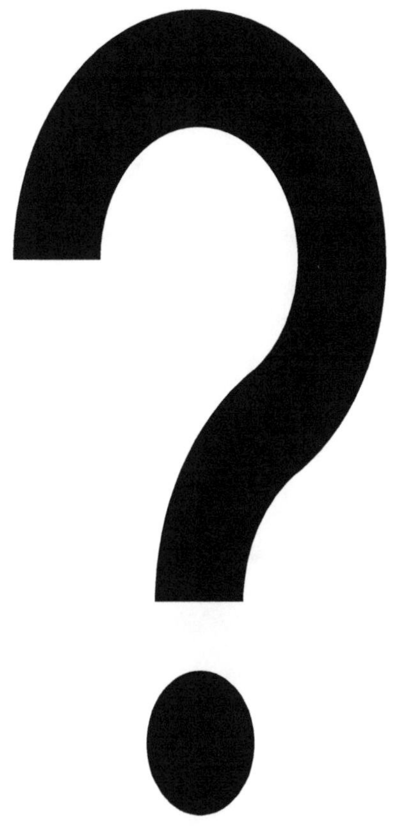

CHILDREN'S BOOK AUTHOR/ AIR FORCE VETERAN

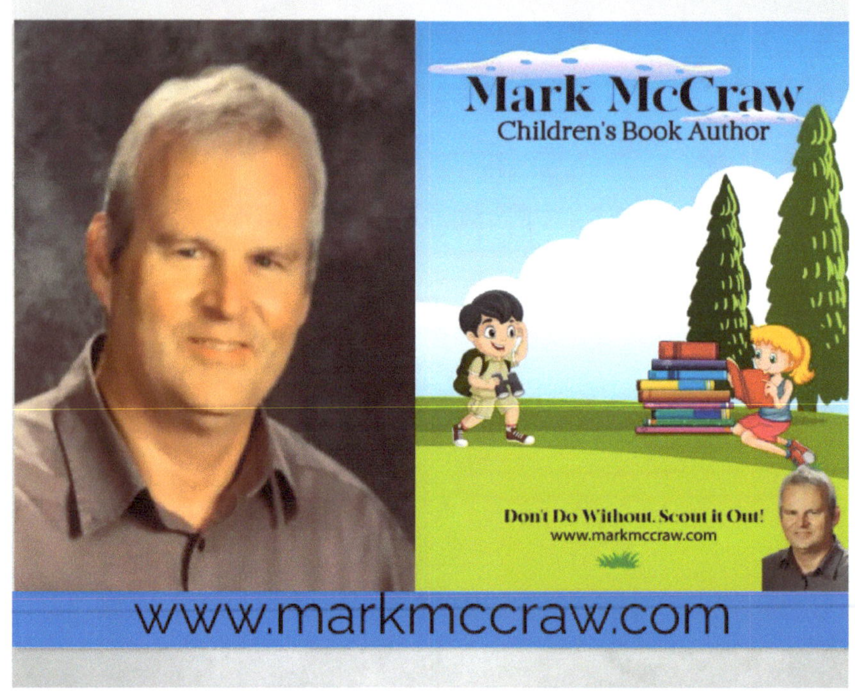

www.MARKMCCRAW.com